I0781608

HOW TO MAKE AND SELL LIP BALM FOR BEGINNERS

Step-By-Step Guide To Crafting, Marketing, And Profiting From Natural, Homemade Mouth Care Products

REMINGTON BRIGGS

DISCLAIMER

Greetings from the world of crafts! Before exploring the fascinating realm of creativity and craftsmanship that this book presents, we would like to make sure that the content is understood and can be clearly understood. This book's contents are meant solely for informational purposes. Although every attempt has been taken to guarantee accuracy and dependability, the material provided should not be used in place of or as a substitute for expert advice. Since every person's path with creating is different, we advise readers to use good judgment and, if necessary, seek out qualified professional guidance.

Crafting calls for imagination, trial & error, and individual interpretation. As a result, depending on personal abilities, tools utilized, and methods employed, outcomes may differ. The concepts, methods, or recommendations offered in this book are not guaranteed to produce any particular results, nor do the writers and publishers of the book. Additionally, it's critical to take safety precautions when working on crafts. Prioritize your own safety and well-being, use the proper tools and equipment, and always adhere to the manufacturer's recommendations.

We urge readers to be aware of their strengths and weaknesses and to experiment, be creative, and enjoy the making process.

TABLE OF CONTENTS

ABOUT THE BOOK

For anyone wishing to enter the world of lip balm creation and entrepreneurship, "How to Make and Sell Lip Balm" is a necessary resource. By explaining the fundamental steps involved in creating lip balm, the introduction establishes a strong basis. It highlights how crucial it is to find high-quality ingredients to guarantee the efficacy and safety of the finished product. Beginners can steer clear of typical mistakes and guarantee a smooth start by selecting the appropriate instruments and following safety procedures. Simple starter recipes are included to give readers a hands-on experience and boost their confidence.

Making a strong base for your lip balm is essential, and this book explores several kinds of bases, including beeswax and shea butter.

It provides thorough directions on how to melt and combine ingredients, guaranteeing the right consistency and texture. Additionally covered are adding moisturizing qualities and storing the base properly, which will assist readers in creating a high-quality product. Scents and flavors: choosing essential oils and fragrances, creating original mixes, and measuring and mixing methods are all covered in this part. Common scenting errors and the significance of allergy and sensitivity testing are also covered.

Customizing lip balm with color gives a unique touch, and this guide offers detailed instructions on safe colorants, how to add color, and how to get the right shade. Another important consideration is packaging, which is covered in the book along with different kinds of containers such as tubes, tins, and jars.

The contents cover filling and sealing techniques, sterilizing and prepping containers, and labeling regulations. Creating a visually appealing product is further aided by creative packaging concepts.

Success is mostly dependent on branding and marketing, and this book walks readers through the process of establishing a brand identity, designing eye-catching labels, and formulating a winning marketing plan. It highlights how crucial it is to communicate with customers on social media and cultivate a devoted clientele.

If you're prepared to sell, creating an online business is made easier with advice on platforms such as Etsy and Shopify, product listing strategies, inventory control, and order processing that guarantees top-notch customer support.

Profitability depends on properly pricing products, and this guide covers cost estimation, competitive pricing, and providing discounts and promotions. Making educated price selections is aided by keeping an eye on market developments and comprehending perceived value. Another option investigated is selling at craft fairs and markets, where tips are provided on event planning, booth setup, and client interaction. To maximize success, the book also provides advice on managing money and following up with attendees after an event.

The book discusses growing a lip balm company by increasing manufacturing and broadening the product offering. It talks about collaborating with shops, controlling expansion, adhering to rules, and guaranteeing sustainable development.

CHAPTER ONE

LIP BALM OVERVIEW

COMPREHENDING THE FUNDAMENTAL PROCEDURE

It's critical to understand the basic steps involved in creating lip balm, which include melting, mixing, and pouring. Start by melting your foundation components in a double boiler. These are usually shea butter, coconut or almond oil, and beeswax. By using two boilers, burning is avoided and even heating is ensured. You can add flavoring and aroma essential oils, as well as any desired colorants, once the components have melted. Make sure all the ingredients are fully incorporated by giving the mixture a good stir.

Then, fill the lip balm containers with the melted mixture. Pots, tins, or tubes can be used, depending on your choice. To prevent clumping, it is crucial to pour the mixture while it is still liquid and warm. Let the filled containers cool to room temperature so they solidify. Usually, this requires several hours. The lip balm is ready to use or sell once it solidifies. Maintaining the quality of your final items requires proper labeling and storage.

Quality testing is the last phase in the fundamental procedure. Make sure your lip balm is effective, consistent, and has a good texture before distributing it. Make sure it feels just right—moisturizing without being overly greasy or harsh. If necessary, make changes to your recipe and record them for use in future batches. The basis for producing lip balm of the highest caliber is laid by this in-depth comprehension of the fundamental procedure.

GETTING GOOD INGREDIENTS

High-quality ingredients are essential to creating exceptional lip balm. Begin by locating beeswax, a naturally occurring thickening and emulsifying substance. To make sure your product is pure, look for beeswax that is organic and devoid of pesticides. Cocoa butter and shea butter work wonders to increase hydration and smoothness. Make sure these butters are unprocessed and additive-free to maintain their original qualities. Additionally essential are carrier oils including jojoba, almond, and coconut oil. Choose organic, cold-pressed oils to preserve their healthful qualities.

Essential oils have several advantages in addition to adding scent. For instance, lavender oil offers relaxing qualities, and peppermint oil can have a cooling impact. To prevent irritating your skin, choose therapeutic-grade, high-quality essential oils. When adding colorants, think about using natural alternatives like beetroot powder or mica powder, which are frequently favored by customers who are searching for natural products and are safer.

It's crucial to buy ingredients from reliable vendors. To confirm the reliability of the source, look for certifications and testimonials. Long-term cost savings can also be achieved by purchasing in bulk, but ingredients must be stored carefully to preserve their quality.

SELECTING THE APPROPRIATE INSTRUMENTS

For lip balm to be produced effectively and consistently, the correct tools must be used.

To safely melt your components without using direct heat, which might harm the oils and waxes, you'll need a double boiler.

You can make do without a double boiler by placing a heatproof bowl over a saucepan of water that is simmering. Because silicone spatulas are easy to clean and heat-resistant, they are perfect for stirring mixtures.

To ensure accuracy and reduce mess, use a small funnel or pipette to carefully transfer the melted balm into containers. Investing in a lip balm filling tray can be beneficial if you're producing lip balm in large quantities. This gadget expedites the procedure and ensures consistency by enabling you to fill numerous tubes or tins at once. Having precise measuring equipment, such as digital scales and measuring spoons, is also necessary to keep your recipes consistent.

Tools for packaging and storage are also essential. To store your bulk supplies fresh and free of contamination, choose airtight containers.

Select visually appealing and easy-to-use containers for your final goods, including colorful tins or twist-up tubes. Labeling equipment, like a printer or label maker, aids in producing labels that meet legal requirements and look professional. Investing in the appropriate equipment can improve the efficiency of your lip balm production process and its overall quality.

SAFETY MEASURES

When creating lip balm, safety is crucial for both you and your clients. To avoid contamination, always begin work in a sanitized and clean atmosphere. To keep yourself hygienic, wash your hands well and think about using a hairnet and gloves. Before using, sterilize all tools and containers by boiling them or applying a disinfectant. This is an essential step in keeping mold and germs out of your lip balm.

Use caution when working with hot substances to prevent burns. Wear gloves that can withstand heat and handle the double boiler carefully. To avoid mishaps, keep kids and dogs away from the work area. To prevent skin sensitivity when using essential oils, make sure you follow the suggested dilution standards.

Since essential oils are powerful, it is best to use them sparingly—a few drops should usually be enough for each batch.

Another important safety precaution is to store your lip balm and its ingredients properly. To avoid melting and deterioration, store completed goods away from direct sunshine in a cool, dry location. To preserve substances' efficacy and freshness, store them in sealed containers.

If you sell your lip balm, make sure to carefully label all of the components to alert customers about any potential allergies. You make sure that both the maker and the user have a safe and delightful experience by following these safety guidelines.

EASY RECIPES FOR NOVICES

To help you become acquainted with the lip balm-making process, start with easy recipes. A simple formula calls for equal amounts of beeswax, coconut oil, and shea butter. Melt the beeswax first, and then stir in the shea butter and coconut oil until well integrated. Take off the heat and savor the aroma with a few drops of your preferred essential oil. Transfer the blend to lip balm vials and let it cool. This recipe yields a moisturizing, silky balm that is simple to work with.

A rich, creamy texture can be achieved with another simple recipe that uses cocoa butter. In a double boiler, mix 2 tablespoons of beeswax, 2 tablespoons of cocoa butter, and 2 tablespoons of almond oil.

Add a spoonful of honey once melted to give it more sweetness and moisture. Add a few drops of essential vanilla oil and stir thoroughly. Transfer to receptacles and let cool. This lip balm smells nice and chocolate and works wonders for dry, chapped lips.

Try this easy recipe for tinted lip balm, which uses beetroot powder to add color. One tablespoon each of jojoba oil, shea butter, and beeswax should be melted. After it has melted, thoroughly mix in 1 teaspoon of beetroot powder. For a revitalizing touch, include a few drops of peppermint essential oil. Transfer into receptacles and allow to cool. This recipe gives your lips a faint hue while also moisturizing them. Using these simple recipes as a starting point can help you gain confidence and proficiency in creating lip balms.

CHAPTER TWO

MAKING THE BASE FOR YOUR LIP BALM

BASE TYPES (SHEA BUTTER, BEESWAX, ETC.)

Making an eye-catching and functional lip balm requires careful consideration of the basis. Because of its inherent emollient qualities, which assist to protect the skin and retain moisture, beeswax is a popular option. It's renowned for its capacity to maintain the lip balm's shape and provide a glossy, smooth finish. In contrast, shea butter is incredibly hydrating and rich in vitamins A and E, which nourish and shield the lips. Its creamy texture gives the lip balm more suppleness. You can also utilize other bases, such as coconut oil or cocoa butter. Coconut oil is light and lends a tropical scent, which enhances the balm's appeal.

Cocoa butter gives the balm a firm texture and a faint chocolate aroma.

Take the intended benefits and consistency into account when choosing a basis. For example, blending shea butter and beeswax produces a well-balanced texture that is moisturizing and firm. Coconut oil can be used to soften the consistency overall, while cocoa butter can be used for extra hardness and a luxurious feel. You can find the ideal balance for your lip balm by experimenting with different base combinations, as each one has special qualities of its own. All skin types can safely and effectively use the finished product because it is made with natural, premium components.

It's crucial to consider the finished product's texture and aroma. The subtle honey aroma of beeswax goes well with a variety of essential oils. The nutty scent of shea butter goes nicely with spicy and sweet scents. Rich and decadent, the chocolate aroma of cocoa butter makes it a popular ingredient in lip balm formulations. Gaining an understanding of each base's unique qualities can help you make lip balm that smells as good as it feels.

METHODS FOR MELTING AND BLENDING

It is imperative to acquire proficiency in melting and blending methods to produce a uniformly smooth lip balm. The components should first be gently heated using the double boiler method.

Put your preferred base—beeswax or shea butter, for example—in a heat-resistant bowl and set it over a saucepan of simmering water. The components will melt gradually and evenly without burning thanks to the indirect heat approach. Until the base is smooth and fully melted, stir it from time to time with a spatula.

You can start adding additional components, such as oils, butter, and essential oils, once the foundation has melted. Add these ingredients little by little, stirring constantly to make sure everything blends evenly. For example, carefully add the coconut oil and essential oils, mixing well until everything is well
blended. This is an essential step in creating a consistent texture and dispersing each ingredient's health benefits throughout the balm.

Once blended, take the mixture off the stove and whisk until it cools a little. By doing this, the components stay together.

While the mixture is still warm and liquid, pour it into lip balm tubes or tins. Before sealing the containers, let the balm cool and firm entirely. Techniques for melting and combining ingredients correctly guarantee a smooth, high-quality lip balm that is prepared for use or sale.

MODIFYING TEXTURE AND UNIFORMITY

It takes considerable tweaking and experimenting to get your lip balm to the ideal texture and consistency. You can soften your lip balm by increasing the proportion of oils or butter in your recipe if it comes out too hard. For example, increasing the amount of shea butter or coconut oil might make the balm creamier and simpler to apply.

On the other hand, adding extra beeswax will firm up the balm and improve its ability to keep its shape if it is too soft and melts readily.

Cooling down can also has an impact on texture. The balm may become gritty if it cools down too rapidly. Let the balm cool gradually at room temperature to prevent this. Another way to keep the mixture smooth while it cools is to stir it every so often. Adding a small amount of vitamin E oil is another tip that helps stabilize the mixture and enhance texture in addition to providing moisturizing benefits.

The secret to getting the perfect texture is to play around with different ingredient and ratio combinations. You might start with a simple recipe and work your way up to the right consistency by gradually adding small amounts of other ingredients. Don't forget to record the proportions utilized in your notes for further usage. You will eventually be able to make lip balm that is both smooth and creamy on the lips and stiff enough to remain solid in the container.

INCORPORATING HYDRATING QUALITIES

If you want your lip balm to have even more moisturizing power, think about adding hydrating and nourishing ingredients. Avocado, almond, and jojoba oils are great options. Jojoba oil is very good at keeping moisture in since it resembles the skin's natural sebum.

Rich in vitamins and fatty acids, almond oil deeply hydrates and relieves dry, chapped lips. Rich in antioxidants and vitamins A, D, and E, avocado oil provides powerful nutrition and defense against environmental harm.

Your lip balm may benefit from the addition of essential oils. Lavender essential oil, for instance, is well-known for its relaxing and restorative qualities, and peppermint essential oil gives lips a revitalizing tingle and increases blood circulation, all of which support healthier lips.

A few drops of these oils can improve your lip balm's moisturizing properties and give it a delightful scent. Just be careful not to use them excessively—essential oils are strong and can irritate skin when used excessively.

For added hydration, you can add substances like honey or aloe vera gel in addition to oils. Since honey is a naturally occurring humectant, it attracts and retains moisture in the skin. Aloe vera gel is an excellent supplement for people who have extremely dry or injured lips because it calms and heals. Your chosen foundation combined with these moisturizing components will produce a lip balm that actively nourishes and heals the lips in addition to providing protection.

MAINTAINING YOUR BASE

It is essential to store your lip balm base properly to preserve its quality and increase its shelf life. Store your lip balm mixture's containers in a cool, dry location away from direct sunlight when they have cooled and formed. The texture, fragrance, and effectiveness of the lip balm can all be negatively impacted by the ingredients' deterioration due to heat and light exposure. A cold, dark cupboard or drawer makes the perfect place to store items.

Consider keeping the base mixture and the finished lip balm separate if you're producing lip balm in large quantities. This enables you to alter tiny batches by adding various ingredients or scents as needed. To avoid infection and moisture absorption, keep the base sealed in a container. To maintain freshness, mark the jar with the preparation date and ingredients. If stored correctly, the majority of handmade lip balms can last up to a year.

Proper storage is even more important for those who sell lip balm because it guarantees that your consumers will receive a high-quality product. Store your inventory in a space with a controlled temperature and make frequent checks for indications of spoiling or separation. Inform your clients on how to store their products to preserve the balm's quality.

CHAPTER THREE

Choosing the correct fragrances and essential oils is vital to creating a lip balm that both soothes the senses and has therapeutic effects. Start by choosing pure, premium essential oils from reliable vendors. Seek oils like lavender, peppermint, and chamomile that are well-known for their safe application in lip care. Think about the benefits of each oil: the soothing powers of chamomile, the refreshing tingle of peppermint, and the calming effects of lavender. To add a pleasing taste, try experimenting with natural flavor extracts like citrus or vanilla.

Steer clear of synthetic perfumes when choosing ones that could hurt delicate skin. Select food-grade, natural extracts that are safe to use on the lips. To make sure there are no dangerous chemicals present, always check the labels. To learn about the strength of each flavor and how it combines with other substances, start with a few fundamental fragrances and flavors. Keep in mind that with small batches of lip balm, strong aromas might be overpowering; less is generally more.

When choosing smells, take your target audience's tastes into account. While robust, energizing perfumes may be preferred by some, others may prefer delicate, subtle odors. Seasonal differences may also play a role; for example, winter odors may be minty, while summer scents may be fruity. You may develop a line of lip balms that satisfy a variety of demands and tastes by experimenting with different essential oils and fragrances.

COMBINING DISTINCT FRAGRANCE COMBINATIONS

It's important to comprehend the interactions between various essential oils to create original smell combinations. Learn the fundamentals of smell classifications, such as citrus, floral, spicy, and woody, first. Try combining oils from several categories to observe how they contrast or complement one another. For example, a common combination of lavender (floral) and lemon (citrus) can be calming and refreshing.

Small test batches are a good way to refine your mixes. To test the scent of each oil before adding it to your lip balm base, mix a few drops of the chosen oils in a carrier oil (such as jojoba). Each oil has three notes that you should pay attention to: the top notes are the first, milder fragrances, the middle notes are the blend's major body, and the base notes are the lingering odors. All three layers are often present in a well-balanced combination for a sophisticated, enticing scent.

Make a note of the ratios utilized in each combination you make in your documentation. This will assist you in duplicating effective mixtures and honing ones that require modification. Never be scared to experiment; sometimes the
most interesting combinations result from pairings you wouldn't expect. For example,

you can make a sweet and refreshing lip balm with vanilla and mint. Through meticulous experimentation and documentation of your mixtures, you will create a distinctive assortment of appealing lip balm fragrances.

TECHNIQUES FOR MEASURING AND MIXING

To consistently produce lip balm of the highest calibre, precise measurement, and mixing are essential. To measure your ingredients properly, use a digital scale. Due to their potency, essential oils and fragrances should only be used sparingly—usually no more than 1% to 2% of the entire mixture. To begin, you should add 5–10 drops of essential oil per ounce of lip balm base, adjusting the amount according to the scent's strength.

Melt the base for your lip balm (beeswax, shea butter, and carrier oils are usually included). To ensure consistent heating and avoid burning, slowly melt these components in a double boiler. After it has melted, take it off the heat source and let it cool down a little before adding your essential oils.

This keeps the medicinal qualities of the oils intact and stops them from evaporating.

To guarantee that the oils are dispersed uniformly, give the mixture a good stir. To prevent contamination, use a stirrer made of glass or stainless steel. The combined product will begin to solidify as it cools, so pour it into lip balm containers soon. Before capping the lip balms, let them cool completely at room temperature. Every batch has a uniform distribution of aroma and a smooth, consistent texture thanks to proper mixing processes.

PREVENTING OFTEN MADE SCENTING ERRORS

Using too much essential oil while scenting lip balm is one of the most frequent blunders made. Overscenting might result in overpowering scents that could irritate others. Always begin with the very minimum advised and increase progressively as necessary. Ignoring the intensity and volatility of various oils is another mistake. Citrus oils, for example, are very volatile and can quickly lose their aroma if they are not measured and blended correctly.

Another mistake is combining smells that are incompatible. Certain essential oils don't mix well and can give off offensive odors when mixed. Try small quantities of every new blend before committing to a larger production run to avoid this. To develop blends that are harmonious and agreeable to the senses, pay attention to how the top, middle, and base notes are balanced.

Finally, poor storage conditions can cause essential oils to lose quality. To keep your oils potent, store them in cold, dry places in dark, airtight containers. The oils may oxidize and lose their scent when exposed to heat, light, or air. You can make sure your lip balms have a constant, delicious aroma that draws in clients by avoiding these typical blunders.

CONDUCTING ALLERGY AND SENSITIVITY TESTING

Making safe, user-friendly lip balms requires testing for allergies and sensitivities. For every new batch of lip balm, start with a patch test.

After applying a tiny amount to the back of the ear or the inner forearm, wait a day to see if there are any effects. This facilitates the identification of any current sensitivity to the essential oils or other components.

When choosing ingredients, take any allergies into account. Allergies to popular oils like coconut or almond may occur in certain persons.

A larger audience can be served by providing a range of formulas, including hypoallergenic alternatives. Make sure that the package for your lip balm has clear labels indicating all contents, including any possible allergies.

Get input from a limited testing pool before the product launch. Request that they report any annoyance or negative reactions. This in-the-field testing offers insightful information on how well your lip balm works on various skin types. You can guarantee that your products are secure and pleasurable for users of all ages by doing thorough testing for allergies and sensitivity.

CHAPTER FOUR

ADDING COLOUR TO YOUR LIP BALM

USE OF SAFE COLOURANTS

It's crucial to use safe colorants when coloring lip balm to guarantee that the finished product is non-toxic and kind to lips. Because they are made especially to be used in items that come into contact with the mouth, food-grade colorants are a great option. Beetroot powder, cocoa powder, and spirulina are examples of natural choices that not only give your lip balm gorgeous colors but also a hint of goodness from nature. Because of its vivid and sparkling qualities, mica powder, a mineral-based colorant that is frequently used in cosmetics, is another safe option.

Choose synthetic colorants that have received FDA approval for use in cosmetics to assure their safety. These colorants are frequently found in store-bought lip cosmetics and have undergone extensive safety testing. FD&C Red No. 40, FD&C Yellow No. 5, and FD&C Blue No. 1 are popular synthetic alternatives. To prevent contamination, always read the label and get colorants from reliable vendors.

Before adding any new colorant to your lip balm, it's crucial to perform a patch test to rule out any adverse responses.

Just dab a little bit of the colored balm onto your wrist, then watch to see if it irritates after a day. This process guarantees that your lip balm will always be mild and safe for all users.

TECHNIQUES FOR INCLUDING COLOUR

You may add color to your lip balm in several efficient ways, each with a different outcome.

One easy method is to blend colorants in powder straight into the melted balm mixture. Melt your base components (beeswax, shea butter, and carrier oils) over low heat to do this. After melting, gradually mix in the powdered colorant, making sure it dissolves well to prevent clumps.

Making a colorant paste and then mixing it into the lip balm recipe is another technique. To make a smooth paste, combine the powdered colorant with a tiny bit of your recipe's oil or liquid.

The melted lip balm foundation can then be combined with this paste to achieve more equal distribution and intense color saturation. When utilizing natural colorants or mica powders that might not dissolve as readily, this technique works very well.

Add liquid colorants, like food coloring or liquid colors, to the melted base drop by drop while stirring continuously.

You may more accurately regulate the color's intensity with this method. Before transferring the mixture into lip balm containers, make sure that the colorant has been thoroughly mixed in.

Try out a few different approaches to see which one best meets your goals as each offers a varying amount of control and finish.

REACHING THE TARGET HUE

Choosing the appropriate colorants and varying their amounts can help you get the ideal shade for your lip balm. To test your colors, start with a tiny batch of lip balm. To start, add a tiny bit of your preferred colorant to the melted base and mix well. To evaluate the color, place a tiny drop on a piece of wax paper or a white surface to observe how it will appear as it cools and solidifies.

Add extra colorant little by little until the desired intensity is achieved if the color is too light. Remember that many colorants—particularly natural ones—may darken or shift slightly as they cool, so before committing to a final hue, make minor tweaks and give the balm some time to set.

 A little goes a long way when it comes to synthetic colorants, so use them sparingly and add more color as needed.

Try blending different colorants to create unique hues. For instance, blending colorants of red and yellow can result in a variety of orange hues, and combining colorants of blue and red can yield a spectrum of purples. Keep track of your ratios and procedures so you can reliably reproduce your preferred shades. It takes some time and some trial and error to get the ideal hue, but the results are worthwhile when you make a one-of-a-kind, customized lip balm.

CHOICES FOR NATURAL AND SYNTHETIC COLOURS

Think about the advantages and features of both natural and synthetic colorants when selecting one for your lip balm. Natural colorants are a safer and more environmentally friendly alternative because they are made from plants, minerals, and other natural sources.

As an illustration, consider using cocoa powder for a rich brown, spirulina for a vivid green, and beetroot powder for a deep red. In addition to giving stunning colors, these colorants frequently have extra skincare advantages including vitamins and antioxidants.

Conversely, man-made synthetic colorants frequently provide more vivid and consistent colors. They come in a greater variety of hues and are usually more stable—that is, they won't deteriorate or change color over time. Because of their dependability and simplicity of usage, synthetic choices such as FD&C and D&C dyes are well-liked in the cosmetics business.

They might, however, contain chemicals that some customers would rather stay away from, particularly those who have sensitive skin or who want natural products.

The decision between natural and synthetic colorants ultimately comes down to your tastes and the demands of your intended audience.

While synthetic colorants provide consistency and adaptability, natural colorants are best for anyone looking for a more delicate and holistic approach.

Both kinds are safe and useful as long as they are purchased from reliable vendors and used by instructions.

SOME ADVICE FOR A BALANCED COLOUR SCHEME

The secret to producing a polished and appealing finished lip balm is to make sure the color is evenly distributed throughout. A good way to go about it is to fully incorporate the colorant into the melted base. While adding the colorant, swirl constantly with a little whisk or a heat-resistant spatula. This guarantees that the color is uniformly distributed throughout the mixture and aids in breaking up any clumps.

If you are using powdered colorants, you might want to prepare a colorant paste in advance by combining the powder with a tiny bit of your recipe's liquid oil.

It is easier and more even to stir this paste into the melted foundation. When adding liquid colorants, do it drop by drop while swirling continuously to keep an eye on the intensity and guarantee uniform blending?

Another way to facilitate the colorant's smoother incorporation is to warm the mixture slightly.

Before transferring the colored mixture into containers, another piece of advice is to strain it through cheesecloth or a fine mesh screen.

This stage guarantees a homogeneous, smooth texture by eliminating any undissolved particles.

To prevent uneven settling, pour the balm into the containers while it's still liquid and warm. These guidelines will help you create a lip balm that is consistently and evenly colored.

CHAPTER FIVE

HOW TO PACKAGE LIP BALM

CONTAINER TYPES (TUBES, TINS, JARS)

The containers you choose for the packaging of your handmade lip balm will determine its final look and functionality. The most popular forms are tubes, tins, and jars; each has certain advantages. The twist-up mechanism of the tubes keeps the balm secure and convenient for usage while on the go.

Tins have a charming vintage appeal and work well with solid balms or tinted formulae because they have a larger surface area for branding and decorating. Contrarily, jars are adaptable and perfect for custom blends or thicker balms because they make it simple for customers to measure out the desired amount.

To preserve the quality and security of your lip balm, make sure your filling containers are clean and sterile. To begin, give them a thorough wash in warm, soapy water and then rinse again. Next, sanitize the containers by immersing them in a solution of water and rubbing alcohol or by using a disinfectant spray. Before filling them with the lip balm recipe, let them air dry fully. This is a crucial step in preventing contamination and extending the product's shelf life.

CONTAINER STERILISATION AND PREPARATION

To preserve cleanliness and product integrity, sterilizing and setting up the containers for your lip balm is an essential stage in the manufacturing process. To start, give your containers a thorough cleaning in warm, soapy water to get rid of any residue or grime. After giving them a thorough rinse, sanitize them by immersing them in a water-rubbing alcohol solution or by using a disinfectant spray. Before using, make sure all surfaces—including caps and lids—are air-dried and sanitized.

After your receptacles have been cleaned and allowed to air dry, arrange them in a tidy and assigned area so that you may fill them. Place them so that simple access is possible during the filling process, guaranteeing effectiveness and avoiding spills or contamination. To reduce confusion and speed up the filling process, name the containers appropriately if you're using multiple kinds of ones. An organized setup improves efficiency and professionalism in your packaging process while also guaranteeing the safety and quality of your lip balm.

METHODS OF FILLING AND SEALING

To fill lip balm containers consistently and attractively, you need to be precise and meticulous in your handling. Use a tiny funnel or pipette to carefully pour the balm mixture into the tubes, making sure not to overfill. If you want to keep the rims looking tidy, wipe off any extra balm.

Tins can be filled with melted balm directly, or for greater control, the surface can be smoothed for a polished appearance with a spatula. To eliminate air pockets from jars, the balm must be gently scooped and pressed using a clean utensil, like a spoon or spatula.

To maintain the freshness and caliber of your lip balm, it is imperative that you properly seal your containers after filling them. To keep tubes hygienic and stop leaks, make sure the caps are snug. To avoid air exposure, tins should be sealed with a lid that fits snugly to provide a tight seal. For extra security, jars can be sealed with inner seals or screw-on lids. Before labeling and packing, check each container for leaks or faulty sealing. You may be confident that your lip balm items are prepared for distribution or sale by using these filling and sealing techniques.

CHAPTER SIX

CREATING A LOGO AND PROMOTING YOUR LIP BALM

ESTABLISHING A PERSONALITY FOR YOUR BRAND

Determining what makes your lip balm special and appealing is the first step in developing a brand identity. Determine who your target market is first. Are you selling to those who are interested in fun, fruity flavors, premium cosmetic products, or eco-conscious consumers? Once you are aware of your target market, create a brand narrative that appeals to them. The purpose, core values, and special advantages of your lip balm should all be highlighted in this narrative. Consider what makes your product unique, such as creative flavors, eco-friendly packaging, or organic ingredients.

Next, pick a name and logo that capture the essence of your business and appeal to your intended audience. While your logo should be straightforward, adaptable, and instantly recognizable, your brand name should be memorable and easy to say.

To produce a professional logo that can be used on all of your branding materials, think about employing a graphic designer. Additionally, the typefaces and colors used for your brand should match the image you wish to convey. For example, natural fonts and earthy tones are ideal for an organic brand, whilst bright, bold colors would be more appropriate for a young, fashionable line.

Lastly, make sure your brand identity is the same on all channels and touchpoints, including your packaging, promotional materials, social media profiles, and website. Customers' faith in the brand is increased by its constancy. To keep your logo, colors, and typefaces consistent, create brand guidelines that specify their appropriate usage.

To stand out in a competitive market and effectively communicate the essence of what your lip balm symbolizes, your brand identity needs to be powerful enough.

CREATING EYE-CATCHING LABELS

Creating eye-catching labels for your lip balm is essential to drawing in potential buyers and providing pertinent product details. Commence with a style that is consistent with your business identity and is straightforward and professional. Your label should have a color scheme that captures the essence of your business and feature your logo and brand name prominently. Utilize top-notch pictures and graphics to give your label a striking appearance. Customers should be able to read and comprehend the design with ease if it is clear and uncluttered.

Apart from being aesthetically pleasing," Make sure this information is presented in a clear and readable manner, using easily readable fonts and colors. Take into account your region's regulatory requirements for cosmetic labeling, including any certificates or warnings that may be required. Gaining your clients' trust can also be accomplished by being open and honest about the benefits of your ingredients.

Lastly, consider the usefulness of your label design. It must be strong enough to resist wear and tear, handling, and exposure to the moisture and oils found in the lip balm.

Select water-resistant and long-lasting materials to avoid fading or peeling. If your brand is committed to sustainability, think about going green. Whether your lip balm container is a tube, tin, or pot, the label should fit snugly to ensure a polished appearance and ease of application. In addition to drawing attention, a well-designed label improves the user experience in general.

FORMULATING A MARKETING PLAN

Creating a lip balm marketing plan entails figuring out the best approaches to connect with and engage your target market. To begin with, gather information about your competition and potential clients' preferences through market research. This study will assist you in determining your product's USPs and the most effective ways to connect with your target market. Establish specific marketing objectives, such as growing your brand's online sales, expanding into new areas, or raising brand awareness.

Next, develop a combination of offline and online channel-leveraging marketing strategies. Create an e-commerce website that is easy to use and optimized for search engines to draw in organic visitors as part of your online marketing strategy. To target particular demographics and interests, spend money on digital advertising through platforms like Google Ads and social network ads. Email newsletters, videos, and blog posts are examples of content marketing that may inform and engage your audience. To reach a larger audience and establish credibility through real testimonials and endorsements, think about forming influencer partnerships.

Investigate offline marketing options such as taking part in regional craft fairs, farmers markets, and beauty expos, where you may present your goods and have in-person conversations with prospective buyers. Give samples to neighborhood salons and boutiques, and incentivize trial purchases with exclusive deals or discounts. Joining trade associations and networking with other small company owners can also offer beneficial exposure and joint venture prospects. These initiatives are combined in a well-rounded marketing strategy to produce a unified and successful plan that promotes expansion and brand awareness.

MAKING USE OF SOCIAL MEDIA

Making good use of social media can greatly expand your lip balm business by raising awareness and fostering interaction with prospective clients. Prioritize the platforms that your target audience uses most frequently when selecting the best ones for your brand. Popular platforms for beauty and personal care products include Facebook, Instagram, and TikTok.

Plan your postings with a content schedule, making sure to include user-generated content, behind-the-scenes glimpses, promotional content, and informative pieces about the advantages of your product and lip care.

Regularly interact with your audience by answering their questions, messages, and mentions. Promote user-generated content by making hashtags, holding giveaways or competitions, and inviting clients to post pictures of them wearing your lip balm. This boosts interaction and offers social confirmation of your product's acceptance. Make use of tools like Instagram Stories and Reels to present customer testimonials, tutorials, and new product launches in a more relaxed and genuine manner.

 Additionally, using live streaming to answer questions, show off how to utilize your products, and engage with your audience in real-time may be quite beneficial.

Social media sites offer analytics tools that can assist you in monitoring the effectiveness of your campaigns and posts. Keep an eye on metrics like click-through rates, follower growth, and engagement rates to find out what material your audience responds to the best. Based on these insights, modify your approach and try out various content kinds, posting schedules, and advertising techniques.

The secret to developing a devoted social media following that converts into actual sales is to be genuine and consistent.

INTERACTING WITH CLIENTS

Maintaining a happy and devoted clientele for your lip balm brand requires active consumer engagement. Start by offering top-notch customer support at every opportunity, including via email, in-person contacts, social media, your website, and email correspondence. Quickly responding to questions and comments demonstrates your appreciation for client input and your dedication to meeting their needs. Personalized communication can improve the customer experience and create a feeling of connection.

Examples of this include utilizing the customers' names in messages and making customized recommendations.

Make it possible for customers to communicate with one another and your brand. Encourage feedback and reviews by providing freebies or discounts as incentives. Organize live chats or Q&A sessions on social media to address frequently asked questions and get comments. Establish loyalty programs that offer points, discounts, or exclusive products as rewards for recurring purchases. Customers are more likely to become repeat customers and brand ambassadors when they feel valued and appreciated.

Seek out and respond to consumer input regularly to enhance your offerings. Distribute surveys to learn more about areas for improvement and consumer satisfaction.

Keep an eye on social media and review platforms to find out what people are saying about your company. Make educated decisions regarding product development, packaging, and customer service procedures by using this feedback. Long-term company success depends on developing trust and loyalty with your consumers, which can be achieved by showing that you pay attention to and care about them.

CHAPTER SEVEN

CREATING AN INTERNET RETAILER

SELECTING A PLATFORM (SHOPIFY, ETSY, ETC.)

Selecting the appropriate platform is essential when opening an online store to sell lip balm. Depending on your demands, platforms like Etsy and Shopify offer different benefits. Because of its intuitive interface and established clientele of people looking for one-of-a-kind and handmade goods, Etsy is ideal for novices. Creating an account is simple, and listing your lip balms will happen fast. But when your company expands, listing and transaction fees on Etsy can mount up.

Conversely, Shopify offers better scalability and customization. It's perfect if you want a more polished store and intend to grow your business. Shopify offers a full range of capabilities, such as inventory management, marketing integrations, and in-depth analytics, but it does charge a monthly subscription fee. Picking a template, personalizing your website, and configuring payment methods are all necessary steps in setting up a Shopify business.

But these can be easily completed with the help of the platform's step-by-step tutorials.

Make sure the platform you select fits both your budget and your business objectives. Use the free trials to examine the characteristics of each choice and determine which one best suits your needs. The secret is to pick a platform that will expand with your company and provide the resources and assistance you require to be successful.

EFFECTIVE PRODUCT LISTING

A product listing's ability to draw in customers and increase sales is essential. Start with crisp photos that highlight the texture and packaging of your lip balm while showcasing it from various perspectives. Capturing the attention of potential consumers can be greatly aided by bright, clear photographs. To help clients visualize using your lip balm in their everyday routine, you should also think about including lifestyle photos of the product in use.

Write enticing product descriptions that go into the ingredients and advantages of your lip balm. To describe the smell, feel, and effects of utilizing your product, use descriptive language. Search terms that prospective buyers might use to find your goods include "organic lip balm," "moisturizing," or "natural ingredients." To set your products apart from the competition, emphasize special features like handmade quality or eco-friendly packaging.

By looking up comparable products on the platform of your choice, you can price your products competitively.

Ensure that your store remains current and enticing to recurring customers by updating your listings frequently to reflect new product variations or seasonal trends.

TAKING CARE OF STOCK

Effective inventory control is necessary to prevent overstocking and stockouts. Begin by meticulously documenting your supplies and final goods.

To keep track of quantities, reorder points, and supplier information, use an inventory management program or spreadsheet. By doing this, you can make sure you never overspend on supplies and that you always have adequate inventory to fulfill client demand.

Establish a mechanism to track sales patterns and modify your inventory as necessary. For instance, schedule the production of extra lip balms in advance if you observe a spike in sales over the holidays or during particular campaigns. To ensure that your records and actual stock match, regularly check your stock levels and perform physical counts. This will help you spot any discrepancies early on.

To guarantee freshness and quality, think about using a first-in, first-out (FIFO) system to make sure older products are sold before fresher ones. In addition to helping you exceed customer expectations, effective inventory management lowers waste and raises overall profitability.

HANDLING PURCHASE ORDERS

Maintaining customer happiness requires you to streamline your order procedure. Send an automated email as soon as an order is placed to confirm receipt and add a thank-you note and anticipated shipment timings. Customers are reassured that their order is being handled effectively by this prompt acknowledgment.

Set up a special packing station with all the resources you'll need, including boxes, bubble wrap, labels, and packing slips, to expedite order preparation. Pack each lip balm carefully to avoid damage during shipping, and add a personal touch with a little sample of another product or a thank-you card. To prevent delivery problems, accurate labeling and accurate shipment information are essential.

Make use of reputable shipping companies and give clients tracking numbers so they can keep an eye on their products. The customer experience can also be improved by processing returns and exchanges quickly and effectively by establishing clear procedures and posting them on your website. Efficient order processing guarantees that clients receive their lip balms on time and undamaged, promoting customer loyalty.

OFFERING TOP-NOTCH CUSTOMER SUPPORT

Providing exceptional customer service can distinguish your lip balm company from rivals.

Be available and quick to respond to consumer questions first. Offer a variety of ways to get in touch, including social media, email, and a form on your website. Aim to react to all concerns within 24 hours, delivering clear and helpful information.

Address client issues with empathy and professionalism. Actively listen to customers' questions and offer solutions, regardless of whether they are regarding ingredients or shipping. Offer quick fixes in the event of an order issue, such as refunds, exchanges, or savings on subsequent orders.

Seek input frequently to make your goods and services better. Promote evaluations and testimonies, and use helpful criticism to make the required changes.

CHAPTER EIGHT

SET YOUR PRODUCT PRICES

FIGURING OUT EXPENSES AND PROFITS

Determine your lip balm's overall cost of production first to set a fair price. This covers the price of tubes or tins for packaging, as well as the cost of raw components such as oils, beeswax, and essential oils. Compiling these costs allows you to see the entire cost per unit.

Next, decide what your ideal profit margin is. A popular strategy is to utilize a percentage for markup. For example, you would price your lip balm at $1.50 if your total cost per unit is $1 and your goal is a 50% profit margin. You can be sure you're covering expenses and turning a profit by using this easy method.

But take into account how much your market is ready to pay, and if needed, modify your margin.

Last but not least, account for any supplemental costs like labor if you're employing help, online shop fees, and promotion. Make sure your pricing plan covers these expenses and yields a respectable return. You may sustain profitability by adjusting prices as necessary by keeping a thorough record of all expenses and analyzing them regularly.

ESTABLISHING COMPETITIVE RATES

Investigate your rivals to find out what identical lip balm items are priced at. Examine local and internet markets to obtain a complete picture. To guarantee that you're comparing like for like, look for products that provide comparable ingredients, quality, and packaging. You can more successfully place your goods in the market with the aid of this study.

After you've established a baseline, think about how your product fits in. You might be able to charge more for your lip balm if it has particular smells or organic components, for example. On the other hand, if your target market is frugal, you may need to reduce your pricing while still making sure your expenses are met. Competitive pricing is about finding a sweet spot where value and affordability combine, not just matching competitors' prices.

Finding the best deal can also be aided by testing out various pricing points. Start with a moderate price and keep an eye on sales. If there is a lot of demand, you could consider raising the price a little. If sales aren't going well, think about offering a promotion to draw in clients. The secret to getting the best deal on your lip balm is to be adaptable and sensitive to consumer input.

PROVIDING SALES AND MARKETING

Promotions and discounts can increase sales and draw in new clients. To begin, schedule seasonal promotions for holidays or other noteworthy occasions. To generate urgency, provide one-time discounts or purchase one, get one free offer. You reach as many people as possible, make sure you promote these offers using email marketing and social media.

Programs for loyalty are yet another successful tactic. Give loyal clients discounts on their subsequent purchases or establish a point system that allows them to accrue prizes for each dollar spent. This creates a devoted consumer base that will probably tell others about your items and encourage repeat business.

Consider the effect that discounts have on your profit margins. Discounts should not reduce your earnings even though they can increase sales. Determine the lowered margin and confirm that the higher sales volume offsets the lower price. Maintaining long-term profitability necessitates careful planning and monitoring of this delicate balancing act.

COMPREHENDING PERCEIVED VALUE

What consumers perceive as the product's value based on considerations other than price is known as perceived value. Prominent components, eye-catching packaging, and a compelling brand narrative can all greatly raise perceived value. In your marketing materials, stressing the advantages of natural components or special formulas can help you defend a premium price point.

Perceived value is significantly influenced by packaging. Invest in sturdy, eye-catching packaging that matches the caliber of your lip balm. This conveys the high-end quality of your product while also grabbing the attention of possible buyers. Eco-friendly packaging can add value and appeal to people who care about the environment.

Reviews and endorsements from customers increase perceived value as well. Urge pleased clients to submit reviews, then prominently display them on your website and social media accounts. Social proof from real-world recommendations increases the confidence of potential buyers in your goods at the pricing you've established.

KEEPING AN EYE ON MARKET TRENDS

Keeping abreast of market developments aids in maintaining the relevance of your pricing approach. Join pertinent online communities; stay up to date on industry news, and sign up for newsletters from professionals in the cosmetics sector. You can modify your offerings and pricing by keeping up with trends in consumer preferences, packaging, and ingredients.

One effective technique for keeping an eye on trends is social media. Look out for what's becoming popular in terms of beauty; platforms such as Instagram and TikTok frequently set trends in this area. Direct feedback on what your audience values and is ready to pay for may also be obtained by interacting with them on these sites.

You may make wise modifications by routinely analyzing your sales data and market trends. If an ingredient gains popularity, think about adding it to your lineup and raising the price to cover the increased benefit. Your lip balm will continue to be competitive and enticing if your pricing strategy is proactive rather than reactive.

CHAPTER NINE

MAKING SALES AT MARKETS AND CRAFT FAIRS

GETTING READY FOR EVENTS

Do extensive research on the event before heading to craft fairs and marketplaces to offer your homemade lip balm. Recognize the target audience, their preferences, the anticipated number of attendees, and the length of the event.

You can use this knowledge to adjust your marketing tactics and product offerings. Next, make a large advance supply purchase. Make sure you have an adequate supply of components, display pieces, packaging materials, and promotional materials (such as business cards or fliers).

To reduce stress at the last minute and maximize productivity, efficiently arrange your desk.

When your materials are prepared, concentrate on designing a visually appealing booth display. When designing your booth, take into account the event's theme and make sure it embodies your business. Showcase your lip balm varieties with eye-catching displays and signage that emphasize their advantages, all-natural ingredients, and distinctive selling features.

Organise and present things in a way that is both visually appealing and easy for customers to browse and choose from. Remember to provide precise pricing information to prevent misunderstandings.

PUTTING UP A VISUALLY APPEALING BOOTH

Getting the right booth setup is essential to drawing clients and increasing sales. Start by deciding on a prominent spot with lots of foot flow within the event area. Arrange a solid tablecloth that matches the colors of your business on it. To make the most of your available area and properly promote your lip balm types, use vertical displays like shelves or stands. Use accent pieces that complement the natural and eco-friendly image of your product, such as lighting, plants, or themed decorations, to create a warm and inviting atmosphere.

Make sure that your merchandise is arranged neatly and is simple for clients to obtain. Assemble related products in groups and properly mark them with summaries that emphasize their salient characteristics.

To provide them with a personal impression of the quality and fragrance of your lip balms, provide samples or testers. To encourage clients to make purchases, use signs and promotional materials strategically to express special offers, promotions, or package deals.

Last but not least, keep your booth tidy and well-maintained during the event to make a good impression on guests.

CUSTOMER INTERACTION

How well you interact with customers can have a big impact on your sales and reputation. Give each guest a warm smile and show genuine concern for their needs. To confidently respond to any queries, be informed on the components, advantages, and uses of your lip balm goods. Actively hear what customers have to say and their preferences; use this data to better personalize product recommendations and enhance upcoming products. Provide tailored advice depending on the skin kinds, inclinations, and any particular worries that your clients may have.

Invite clients to test samples or testers and offer frank comments. Make use of this chance to inform them of the ingredients used, emphasizing characteristics that are sustainable and natural to appeal to eco-conscious customers. Talk about your brand's history and your love of making high-quality lip care products to connect with clients on a deeper level than just business. Gather social media handles or contact details for the next marketing campaigns and follow-up correspondence. Express gratitude to consumers for their support and urge them to tell others about your lip balm line.

MANAGING PAYMENTS

For a flawless client experience, the payment process must be streamlined. Provide a variety of payment methods, including cash, credit/debit cards, and electronic ones like payment applications or mobile wallets. Each product's price should be prominently shown, along with any relevant discounts or promotions. To handle transactions quickly and effectively, use a mobile card reader or point-of-sale (POS) system that is dependable and secure. For inventory management and financial tracking, provide receipts or invoices for every purchase and make sure that sales data is accurately recorded.

Make sure you have backup payment choices or manual transaction methods in place in case of any technological difficulties.

If necessary, provide your staff with training on managing payments and responding to questions or issues from customers about exchanges, refunds, or prices. Throughout the payment process, act with professionalism and openness to make sure consumers are comfortable and happy with their purchases. As a thank you for their business, offer to help pack or move their belongings as a demonstration of your superior customer service.

POST-EVENT FOLLOW-UPS

Your attempts to engage customers don't end when a craft fair or market event ends. To foster relationships and promote repeat business, follow up with participants and possible leads. Thank them personally via emails or texts for visiting and showing interest in your lip balm line. As a thank you and enticement for more purchases, include a code or special offer.

Get consumer feedback regarding their impressions of your lip balm items and their experience attending the event? Make use of this input to pinpoint areas that need work and hone your marketing plans for upcoming events. To keep your business visible and interact with customers who found it at the event, be active on social media. To keep people interested in your products and engaged, include behind-the-scenes content, consumer testimonials, and highlights from the event. After the event, keep up the relationship-building with consumers to promote brand advocacy and loyalty for your lip balm.

CHAPTER TEN

GROWING YOUR LIP BALM COMPANY

EXPANDING THE SCOPE OF YOUR PRODUCT OFFERING

Creativity is your best friend when it comes to expanding your lip balm business. Start by coming up with novel flavors or combinations that will suit a range of consumer tastes. Consider using seasonal variants, such as pumpkin spice in the fall or mint in the summer.

Investigating niche markets that appeal to health-conscious consumers, such as those for vegan or organic lip balms, is an additional strategy. Remember packaging: distinctive styles or environmentally friendly materials can make your products stand out on store shelves.

It's time to test out new products once you've made your decision. To get input from friends, family, or focus groups, do small-scale trials. Before going into full-scale manufacturing, use this feedback to improve your packaging and recipes. Recall that expanding your product line's diversity means catering to the varied wants and preferences of your target market, not just offering more options.

It's time to market your products wisely now that you have a variety of them ready. Showcase your newest products at craft festivals, neighborhood markets, and social media. Draw attention to the distinctive qualities of each product and how they satisfy a range of consumer preferences. Strategically expanding your product line will help you reach a larger clientele and generate more revenue.

Growing your lip balm business requires you to scale up production to keep up with demand. To commence, evaluate your existing production capability and pinpoint opportunities for enhancement. This could entail making larger equipment investments, streamlining the production process, or recruiting more workers. Simplifying processes without sacrificing the reliability and quality of the final product is the aim.

In terms of increasing productivity, automation can be revolutionary. Seek to automate monotonous processes such as product labeling or container filling. This lowers the possibility of mistakes while also increasing efficiency. To free up internal resources, think about contracting out some activities, like packaging or shipping, to other companies.

When increasing output, quality control is crucial. To make sure that every batch satisfies your requirements for texture, smell, and shelf life, put strict testing procedures in place. Keep a close eye on production data such as defect and yield rates to spot areas that could use more optimization. Strategic production scaling allows you to fulfill increasing demand without sacrificing product quality.

COLLABORATING WITH STORES

The reach and visibility of your lip balm business can be greatly increased by partnering with stores. Investigate possible retail partners who share the same values as your target market and brand.

Make a strong pitch to them that emphasize the advantages of working together as well as the special features of your products. Stress how your lip balms can improve their product line and draw in new clients.

Successful retail collaborations require careful negotiation of favorable terms. Think about things like cost, terms of payment, and marketing assistance. To help retailers properly present their products in-store or online, be ready to supply them with marketing materials, product samples, and training materials. Developing trusting bonds with retailers can result in long-term collaborations and mutual success.

Work together with merchants on marketing campaigns that will boost revenue and brand awareness. Co-branded advertising, new product releases, and in-store displays are a few examples of this. To keep refining your partnership plans, track sales performance and get input from retail partners. Strategic partnerships with retailers allow you to reach new markets and grow your clientele.